The Do's and Don'ts of the Keto Diet

The Must-Have Keto Foods

The Do's and Don'ts of the Keto Diet

By Troy Gorham

The Do's and Don'ts of the Keto Diet

By reading any document, the reader agrees that under no circumstances are we responsible for any losses, direct or indirect, which are incurred as a result of use of the information contained within this document, including – but not limited to errors, omissions, or inaccuracies.

Table of Contents

The Do's and Don'ts of the Keto Diet

Chapter #1: Introduction

Are you considering the keto diet? This diet is one of the latest trends, although it's actually been around for many years. Because of this, it's not really a "trend" at all. Instead, it's more like an effective diet with plenty of research behind it. None of this really explains what the keto diet is and how to follow it, which is why you're here, right? We'll explain all of the basics of this diet, as well as what you should and should not be eating while on it.

The Keto Diet Can Change Your Life

If you've struggled with weight loss in the past and haven't had much success, then you need to try the keto diet. Once your body goes into ketosis and your fat stores begin to disappear, you'll see just how effective this diet is. In fact, if you follow it correctly, you'll even have more energy and a clearer mind.

Do you want to learn more about this effective diet? If so, keep reading!

Chapter #2: What Is the Keto Diet?

Let's define the keto diet in simple terms. Basically, it involves eating few carbohydrates and avoiding foods that are high in sugar. Although you might think that the diet is no carb, it is

The Do's and Don'ts of the Keto Diet

actually low carb. This is a big difference because you're allowed to eat carbs, just in very small amounts.

Sending Your Body Into Ketosis

The purpose of following the keto diet is to send your body into a state of ketosis. What's ketosis? It's when your body burns off its fat stores, causing you to lose weight. You've probably noticed that the word "keto" is very similar to "ketosis." This is where the name of the diet comes from. However, there's a third related word that you need to know – ketones.

When your body is in ketosis, it produces these ketones. They are formed in the liver from the fat that you lose while following the diet and being in ketosis. Have you followed this so far? If not – you eat a diet that's low in carbs and sugars. This sends your body into ketosis (which is essentially a metabolic state), where the fat stores are processed for energy. The fat is processed through your liver in the form of ketones.

The important points here are that you lose weight as your fat stores vanish. This is more effective than most diet and exercise plans since the keto diet directly affects your body fat. As you lose this weight, you'll have more energy and will able to think more clearly, since the ketones become fuel for your body and your brain.

That sounds simple enough, right?

Macros and Micros

When you're on the keto diet, tracking your macronutrient intake is essential. You need to know exactly how many grams of fats, protein, and carbohydrates you're eating each day. Your meals need to be properly portioned in order to receive the most benefits from the diet. This is done by tracking your macronutrients (also known as macros) and your micronutrients (shortened to micros.) There are a number of apps that can help you with this, as long as you enter your recipes and portion sizes into them.

However, you also need to know what macros and micros are.

Macros

These are the nutrients that you need to focus on. There are three of them that fall into this category – proteins, fats, and carbohydrates. While on the keto diet, you want to eat a lot of

The Do's and Don'ts of the Keto Diet

first of them (proteins), some of the second (fats), and not very much of the third (carbohydrates.) As we've already mentioned, this diet is low-carb, not no-carb, so you'll be eating a very, very small amount of carbohydrates each day.

Micros

Your micros are things like vitamins and minerals. You need to have a healthy balance of them in order to feel good and keep your body in great condition. Things like Vitamin A, Vitamin C, and Vitamin D are important, as are minerals like magnesium, potassium, and calcium. Since you won't eat much dairy (if any at all) while on the keto diet, you'll need to include some supplements that will fill in any gaps in your overall nutrition. The key here is to feel better while losing weight, not to eat an unhealthy balance of foods that could make you sick.

The Keto Flu

Speaking of "getting sick," you've probably heard rumors of the keto flu. This is indeed something that exists, but it's not a real flu that's caused by a virus or bacteria. Instead, it simply feels like you have the flu, because you won't have any energy and will feel poorly.

The Do's and Don'ts of the Keto Diet

The keto flu tends to strike in the first week that you're on the diet. It's your body's way of letting you know that you're detoxing from carbohydrates and sugars. Some of the symptoms include things like nausea, a headache, dizziness, and plenty of aches and pains. You may not be able to focus, and you'll generally feel very bad for between 24 and 48 hours (or longer, depending on how many carbs and sugary foods that you ate before starting the diet.)

Thankfully, you won't have any of the traditional flu symptoms like a runny nose, coughing, sneezing, or stuffiness. This tends to make the keto flu a bit more bearable.

If you want to treat the keto flu so that you can keep functioning without letting it get to you too badly, then you just need to drink plenty of water and take some nutritional supplements, such as those containing potassium and magnesium. You can also eat salty foods, and if the flu makes you feel very bad, you can eat a tiny amount of carbs. As long as you stay in ketosis and keep that amount of carbs low, then you will feel better after a short time.

However, you can choose to not treat the keto flu at all, since you know that you'll be over it very quickly – and then you'll be well on your way to losing weight, burning fat, and having plenty of energy. The keto flu is just a small bump in the road. It's no cause for alarm, and it's certainly not a reason to stop following the diet.

History of the Keto Diet

The keto diet may not have become popular until recently (although it saw a surge in popularity in the 1990s), but it actually dates back thousands of years to Ancient Greece.

Let's travel back in time (at least on paper) to 600 BCE. There were two Greek physicians (using the term loosely) who experimented with what they called a fasting diet. It consisted of eating mainly meat, while not eating a lot of bread. Those physicians, Galen and Erasistratus, put people with seizure disorders on this diet and saw some success. However, nothing was really done about it for several thousand more years.

Jumping ahead to the 20th century, 1911 to be precise, is when scientists and doctors discovered that the ideas put forth by Galen and Erasistratus were valid. They began putting patients with epilepsy (by now it had a name) on a low-carb diet. When their seizures were reduced in number, these scientists knew that they had something useful on their hands.

The Do's and Don'ts of the Keto Diet

A mere ten years later, ketone bodies were discovered. There are two physicians who are credited with moving the diet forward in a scientific manner. The first is Rollin Woodyatt who actually discovered those ketone bodies. He was doing research on diabetes when he found them. The second researcher, Russel Wilder, worked for the Mayo Clinic. He is the person who actually coined the term "ketogenic diet."

In between 1921 and the 1960s, very little noteworthy research was done on the diet. However, in the 1960s, medium-chain triglycerides (also known as MCTs) were discovered to have an effect on those ketone bodies. The researchers involved in this study were looking at the ways to prevent people with epilepsy from having seizures, without having to put them on the harsh, side-effect filled medications that existed at the time. These days, MCTs are an important part of every keto diet.

Finally, in the 1990s, bodybuilders discovered the diet and found that if they stayed on it, they burned off their body fat in the form of energy, while producing lean muscle mass at the same time. The diet hasn't changed much since then, although many people – not just bodybuilders – have experienced its benefits.

The Do's and Don'ts of the Keto Diet

Why have we told you about this brief history of the diet? The answer is simple – because something that's been around for this long is more than just a flash in the pan or a trend. It's actually something that people have been following for thousands of years, off and on. That longevity counts for something.

Health Issues That the Keto Diet Can Help

Did you know that the keto diet can help certain health conditions? Sure, you're more than likely using it to lose weight, but know the conditions that it can treat lends some credence to the diet – and it can help you detract any naysayers. They include:

- Alzheimer's Disease
- Epilepsy
- Multiple Sclerosis
- Parkinson's Disease
- Polycystic Ovarian Syndrome (PCOS)
- Autism
- Metabolic Syndrome/Pre-diabetes

The Do's and Don'ts of the Keto Diet

Is There Anyone Who Shouldn't Follow the Keto Diet?

Although no one should embark on a new diet without checking with their doctor first, if you're diabetic, have high blood pressure, or are pregnant or breastfeeding, then you should avoid this diet – at least until your doctor gives you the okay.

Now That You Understand The Keto Diet

Hopefully, you understand the keto diet a little better than you did in the past. You know how to follow it and you understand what macros and micros are. You're informed about the keto flu. The history of this diet is no longer a mystery. You also know what types of medical conditions it can treat, as well as the ones that may prevent you from following it. Now it's time to talk about food.

Chapter #3: Best Keto Foods to Eat

Now that you know more about the keto diet itself, it's time to cover what you should be eating in order to follow it properly. There are a number of good foods that you can include in your diet, all of which will help you reach and stay in ketosis while ingesting the proper amounts of macros and micros.

Dark Chocolate

Let's start off with a universal favorite – dark chocolate. The key here is the word "dark." You need to keep an eye on the overall cocoa content and remember that the higher it is, the better. If you find a dark chocolate that's more than 80%

cocoa, then you're safe. Anything lower has a higher sugar content, as well as more additives, and it could send you out of ketosis.

With that said, you shouldn't incorporate a lot of dark chocolate into your diet. You need to treat it as if it were, well, a treat! Plus, you don't have to eat it plain, in bar form, unless you want to. There are plenty of keto friendly dessert recipes that include dark chocolate.

Dairy

Generally, people on the keto diet tend to avoid many "classic" forms of dairy, like milk. Instead, they go for things with a higher calcium content, such as hard cheeses, plain yogurt (watch the sugar content), and cottage cheese. All of these foods are low-carb and low in sugar, so they meet the needs of the diet while allowing you to get in those important micros, such as calcium and Vitamin D.

If you're worried that one of them might contain too many carbohydrates or sugars, just read the labels. You could end up being pleasantly surprised.

Red Meat

The Do's and Don'ts of the Keto Diet

Red meat is one of the staples of the keto diet since you do need to eat a lot of protein and incorporate some healthy fats into your meals. This means that you'll have to get used to learning about the different cuts of red meat in order to determine which ones will work best.

For example, you want to stick to things like roasts and steaks, both of which contain plenty of the right nutrients. If you do decide to use ground beef for a meal, make sure that you purchase the one with a 90/10 ratio of meat to fat. You don't want to go below that, as the fat content can be too high.

On top of this, if you can purchase red meats that come from cattle that have been fed an organic grass diet from a farm that avoids feeding them a lot of processed grains and antibiotics, then go ahead and do so. These meats are better for you and allow you to follow your keto diet to the letter.

Poultry

Poultry, including chicken, duck, goose, and even Cornish game hens, are another staple of the keto diet. Just like with the red meat that you purchase, you do want to try to find birds that have been fed an organic diet and have been allowed to graze. The ones that are raised in cages and treated inhumanely may taste okay, but they are not as good for you as the other ones.

In general, poultry is easy to make and comes in a number of different formations. You can include dark meat, like legs and thighs in your meals one day, and then chicken breasts the next. Since you do need some fat content in your diet, you don't have to worry as much about removing the skin before you cook it. Ideally, your meals should consist of plenty of chicken and some beef (as described above.)

Seafood

Seafood rounds out the list of meats that you can eat while on the keto diet. Seafood, in general, is incredibly good for you, as it contains plenty of vitamins and minerals. It's also very low in carbohydrates (basically, everything from these bodies of water is low-carb), and there are plenty of options, which means that you'll never get bored of eating the same thing over and over again. You need to incorporate plenty of seafood into your diet. Some options include:

- Shrimp
- Mussels
- Claims

The Do's and Don'ts of the Keto Diet

- Tuna (fresh, frozen, or canned)
- Crabs
- Salmon
- Sardines
- Striped Bass
- And more

Eggs

It's impossible to list the foods that you should eat while on the keto diet and not include eggs. Not only do eggs contain a lot of protein, but they are also very low in carbohydrates. In general, one single egg (no matter the size) contains a mere 1 gram of carbs. This means that you incorporate them into your diet in any number of different ways.

Some people on the keto diet have eggs for breakfast, while others tend to eat them for lunch (you can fry one and toss it on a salad), or even for dinner. If you can, stick with brown eggs, or find ones from a local organic farm. They might cost more, but they are much better for you – and they taste better as well.

Vegetables

The Do's and Don'ts of the Keto Diet

You can't a proper diet and get the right amounts of macros and micros without eating a lot of vegetables. While some are high in carbohydrates (like potatoes and beets), most of them are not, which makes them a good side dish for every meal. You can make yourself a nice salad full of green leafy vegetables like kale and spinach (and even lettuce), or steam up some broccoli or Brussels sprouts.

However, you do need to keep in mind that when you're eating salad, you shouldn't douse your vegetables with a sugar-filled salad dressing. No matter how much you like ranch dressing or creamy Caesar, you need to steer clear of them. Instead, top your salads with oil-based dressings (read the labels first), or just use a drizzle of coconut oil instead.

Coconut Oil

Speaking of coconut oil, you'll need some sort of oil to cook with. While you could use a simple olive oil, you should actually aim for something with a bit more of a nutritional punch, like coconut oil.

What's so great about coconut oil? This substance is actually considered a superfood because it has plenty of vitamins, minerals, and antioxidants. It even contains MCTs, which we

The Do's and Don'ts of the Keto Diet

discussed (briefly) earlier. It's a great – and very healthy – alternative to things like butter and traditional cooking oils.

Avocados

If you're on the keto diet, then you need to find a way to incorporate avocados into your meals. These green fruits are very high in healthy fats and contain plenty of vitamins and minerals. Plus, you can eat them in many different ways – as long as you steer clear of guacamole. This dip and topping usually contain tomatoes, which are high in sugar.

Greens Powder

Many people on the keto diet make themselves smoothies in the morning with greens powder. This powder is exactly what it sounds like – it's green – and it comes in powder form. You can add a scoop of it to your smoothies, or just dissolve it in a glass of water and drink it in the morning. It tends to contain a number of important vitamins and minerals and is a great way to ensure that you're eating all of the right micros.

Chapter #4: Easiest Keto Foods to Find and Prepare

While the number of foods that should be included in the keto diet may seem kind of daunting, what matters is that many of them easy to locate and prepare. You should be able to find many of them at your local grocery store, and cooking (or baking) them is easy. If you need some meal inspiration, but don't have a lot of time to prep and cook your meals, then you need to consider some of the options below.

The Do's and Don'ts of the Keto Diet

Eggs and Greens

Some of the easiest meals to make consist of eggs and greens. Simply warm up a bit of coconut oil in a pan and then fry up your eggs in it. You can scramble them as well, as long as you add water instead of milk to the mix in order to fluff them up a bit. In a separate pan, also with some coconut oil, warm up a helping of kale and spinach. Serve the cooked eggs on top of the greens. You can even shred a bit of hard cheese and place it on top. This meal works well for breakfast, lunch, and even dinner.

Yogurt and Fruit

Although you do need to be careful and not eat too much sugar, you can get away with including a small amount of it in a keto-friendly meal. Start by choosing a tasty, unseasoned (read: plain) yogurt that hasn't had a lot of sugar added to it. A Greek yogurt is a good option. Then, sprinkle a few berries on top (blueberries, strawberries, and other types of berries work well), and eat. This is a quick and easy breakfast, and it also makes a good afternoon snack.

The Do's and Don'ts of the Keto Diet

The trick to making this keto-friendly is, as we've already mentioned, choosing a plain yogurt and only adding a few – no more than five or six – berries. Too much sugar can send you out of ketosis.

Baked Chicken Quarters

Chicken quarters (which consist of a leg and a thigh attached to each other) contain a lot of dark meat. This means that they are full of healthy fats and protein, as well as flavor. Baked chicken is incredibly easy to make since all that you need to do is drip some oil on a baking pan to keep the chicken from sticking and then sprinkle on some seasonings. A mix of salt, pepper, garlic, and even paprika works well. You can also include some dried chives, green onion, parsley, and basil. Bake the chicken at 400 degrees Fahrenheit until it's at an internal temperature of 165 degrees. This usually takes around 50 minutes, although it depends on your oven.

Serve your baked chicken with cauliflower rice and a salad.

Cauliflower Rice

Since you need to steer clear of grains like traditional rice (even brown rice, Jasmine Rice, and other forms have too many carbohydrates) your best bet is to make rice from a

The Do's and Don'ts of the Keto Diet

head of cauliflower. You'll need the aforementioned cauliflower, as well as a food processor.

Wash the cauliflower well and break into chunks. Place them in the food processor and pulse them until they are in small bits that resemble grains of rice. Then, you need to heat a pan (with a bit of coconut oil dribbled on) and put the cauliflower rice on it. Season it with some salt and pepper, although if you want to, you can add in some additional spices as well. (One of the best things about spices is that they are very keto-friendly.) A bit of dried onion and some chives work well with the cauliflower.

Once the bits of "rice" are soft and tender, they are ready to eat and serve. This makes a great side dish for the chicken thighs recipe listed above, although you can serve it with just about any other meat as well.

Salad

Nothing works better as a side dish quite like a green salad. There are so many different things to add – all of which are very keto-friendly – that you have a lot of options. You might not even eat the same salad twice in a row!

The Do's and Don'ts of the Keto Diet

Start with a bed of greens, such as kale, spinach, and/or one of the many different types of lettuce. (There are literally dozens of different types of lettuce.) Add in some carrots and radishes, as well as a few pieces of onion, and then serve with a side of olive oil or coconut oil. You can even create an olive oil blend by placing a few pieces of garlic or basil it in for around 24 hours before serving. This will give your salad a little more flavor.

Tuna Steak

If you like seafood, then this is a great entrée. Tuna, in general, is great for people on a keto diet, as it's very high in protein, contains plenty of good fats, and even has some antioxidants and other micros. With that said, there's a fear of ingesting lead along with your tuna, so you may not want to eat it every single day. Instead, have it once a week or so.

Prepare your tuna steak by drizzling some coconut oil on a baking sheet or pan. Pour a little on the tuna as well. Then, follow this with some seasonings. Lemon juice, which is keto-friendly in small amounts, and some salt and pepper are typically all that you need. Bake the tuna steak at 350 degrees Fahrenheit for around 20 minutes or half an hour until it's tender and flaky. Serve your tuna steak with a salad and some cauliflower rice.

Make Pot Roast in Your Crockpot

Traditionally, pot roast is served alongside carrots and potatoes, but you'll need to limit your intake of them in order to remain in ketosis. Instead, serve the meat plain, with some of the "sauce" that it's cooked in. Of course, as we already mentioned, cauliflower rice and a salad work well with it.

Place your pot roast in the bottom of your crockpot. Sprinkle it liberally with Montreal Steak Seasoning, as well as salt and pepper. Add in an onion, chopped, and some garlic. Pour in two cups of beef broth, as well as two tablespoons of Worcestershire sauce.

Set your crock pot on high for six hours. When the meat is falling apart, it's done.

As you can see, there are plenty of easy keto-friendly recipes out there. These are just a few examples to get you started.

Chapter #5: Foods to Avoid

Of course, there are plenty of foods that you need to avoid while following the keto diet. If you incorporate these items into your meals, you risk sending your body out of ketosis, thus making it less likely that you'll experience all of the positive side effects of the diet. Here are the foods that you need to steer clear of.

Grains

Grains, which include things like wheat and rice, are very high in carbohydrates. You'll notice that a lot of the more complicated keto recipes include substitutes for grains, such as almond flour. You want to experiment with these alternatives if you want to make your own baked goods.

The Do's and Don'ts of the Keto Diet

Alternative flours are great options for rolls, cakes, bread, and more.

Of course, it needs to be emphasized here that you need to avoid anything that is made with these traditional grains. This means that you can't have loaves of bread from the grocery, bakery rolls, or even cakes and cupcakes. Cookies tend to be out as well unless you've made them yourself from an alternative flour.

Rice is out, too, but we've already mentioned that. It's too high in carbs.

Legumes and Beans

Like grains, legumes and beans are high in carbs. This means that they shouldn't be included in a keto diet. You might be able to get away with small amounts of them, but they do need to be included sparingly, and as long as your other macros are okay. Generally, you're allowed between 30 and 50 grams of carbohydrates a day, so if you haven't had any others that day, you can have some beans or legumes with your meal.

Sugar-filled Foods

The Do's and Don'ts of the Keto Diet

The entire point of the keto diet is to stay in ketosis, which means that foods that contain a large amount of sugar are general out. This is one of the toughest things for people starting the diet to give up, but it must be done. You can find sugar in the following things:

- Chocolate-based candies
- Non-chocolate candies
- Cookies
- Cupcakes
- Cake
- Frosting
- Granola bars
- Soda
- Certain coffee-based beverages
- Sauces (BBQ sauce, spaghetti sauce, ketchup)
- Canned baked beans
- Processed fruit juices
- Sports drinks that also have electrolytes
- Milk
- Processed iced tea
- Cereals
- Canned and powdered soups
- Cream-based salad dressings
  - Flavored milk

- Ice cream
- Dessert bars

And so on. There are a lot of things out there that contain sugar as an additive!

Fruit

Fruit tastes good. It also contains a lot of sugar, which makes it bad for people on a keto diet. You need to avoid fruit almost entirely. This means that you also have to avoid fruits that most people think of as vegetables, including tomatoes and cucumbers.

With that said, you are allowed a few berries a day, as long as your overall sugar levels are low. The recipe included in the previous chapter includes some with a helping of yogurt.

Alcohol

Did you know that alcohol contains a lot of sugar? During the fermenting process, the added grains (another no-no for people on a keto diet) turn into sugars, giving these beverages their signature tastes and adding to their alcohol content. For all of these reasons, alcoholic beverages of all kinds need to be avoided while on a keto diet.

The Do's and Don'ts of the Keto Diet

Plus, if you're familiar with the term "beer belly" then you already know to stay away from fermented, alcoholic beverages while trying to lose weight in general.

Milk and Butter

Although you can have other dairy products, including things like eggs, hard cheeses, cottage cheese, and plain yogurt, you need to avoid milk and butter when on a keto diet. Both are high in sugar, and they also contain some carbohydrates.

Since you shouldn't have cereal while on this diet, milk is easy to avoid. Coconut oil makes a good butter substitute.

Processed Foods

Many of the processed foods that you find on store shelves contain hidden carbohydrates and sugars. Just look at the labels on the packaging. If you see things like "high fructose corn syrup," you're looking at pure sugar. Always read the labels. However, you're better off steering clear of premade foods, even those that claim to be low in calories and "keto friendly."

Starches

The Do's and Don'ts of the Keto Diet

In addition to everything else on the list, you need to avoid starchy foods, like potatoes and sweet potatoes. They contain a lot of carbohydrates and even some sugars.

As you can see, there are a number of foods that need to be avoided in order to stay in ketosis.

Chapter #6: Testing for Ketosis

The Do's and Don'ts of the Keto Diet

The goal of everyone on the keto diet is to send their bodies into a state of ketosis. If you've been following along so far, then you know that this the point where your body begins using up those fat stores, sending them to the liver, which turns them into ketones. The real question is: how can you tell when you're in ketosis? There are several things to look for.

Check Your Breath

Did you know that ketones can change the way that your breath smells? They can indeed! You might notice some changes to your breath, including a slightly sweetened odor. It could appear as an unusual taste in your mouth, although some people just smell it on their breath.

(Fun fact: ketones can change the smell of your urine as well.)

Ketones can turn into acetones, which appear in the mouth in the form of that sweet, slightly fruity smell. Don't confuse these acetones with the ones in your nail polish remover – those are quite different. Instead, the acetones produced by the ketones are a natural bodily function that indicates that you are indeed in ketosis. Your diet efforts have been worthwhile!

Test Your Blood

The Do's and Don'ts of the Keto Diet

Another way to check the levels of ketones in your system is by using a blood monitor. You'll able to find a ketosis monitor in many different stores. They work in the same way as the glucose monitors sold for people with diabetes – you simply prick your skin, squeeze out a blood drop, and then run it through the monitor. The only difference is that instead of checking your blood's glucose levels, you're actually measuring the levels of beta-hydroxybutyrate (BHB) that are in your bloodstream.

Beta-hydroxybutyrate (BHB) is yet another ketone; one that appears in your blood. If high enough levels are present (and the monitor will let you know), then you are in ketosis.

Use a Breath Indicator or Urine Test Strips
If the thought of testing a drop of blood makes you squeamish, then you need to use one of these additional methods of measuring the ketones in your system. We've already mentioned the fact that the smells of your breath and urine will change when you're in ketosis thanks to the additional acetones produced by your body. There are monitoring devices that can check this for you. With the breath indicator device, you just blow into it and you'll receive a response about whether or not you're in ketosis. The urine strips are just

as easy to use, although they are a little messier. As you can imagine, you need to urinate into the included container and then dip the strip into it. If you're in ketosis, the strip will change colors.

You Lose Weight

Sometimes you can tell that you're in ketosis without even using any of the monitoring devices. Instead, you just need to look in the mirror. If you've lost weight and are clearly skinnier, then the diet is working – and you're more than likely in ketosis.

However, the length of time that you've been following the diet matters here as well. If you've been on it for only a week, then the weight loss that you've experienced could just be general water weight or the effects of cutting back (extremely) on the amount of sugar and carbs that you eat. If you're like more people, then both of these are things that you've indulged in before starting the diet. Most people on the keto diet see an immediate weight loss for these reasons.

But, if you've been on the diet for a longer period of time and are still experiencing weight loss, then you're in ketosis. It could take a few weeks before you experience this type of

The Do's and Don'ts of the Keto Diet

weight loss, which comes from losing those annoying fat stores that have plagued you.

Your Appetite Is Smaller

Once you're in ketosis, you'll notice that your appetite is smaller than it has been. Although this happens with many diets, especially as you begin to adjust to eating smaller portions, it's particularly noticeable in people who are following the keto diet.

There are several reasons why you'll be less hungry while on the keto diet. The first is that the ketones in your brain are reducing your appetite, thus making you less hungry. This isn't a bad thing at all – it just means that you're on the right track. In addition to this, you're eating a lot more vegetables (the right kinds of vegetables that is) which contain plenty of fiber. The more of them that you eat, the fuller that you'll feel for a longer period of time. As a result, the food that you eat is digested slower (as it should be) making you feel less hungry.

Once you're in ketosis, you'll notice this side effect.

You Have More Energy and Can Focus Better

The Do's and Don'ts of the Keto Diet

We've mentioned this earlier as one of the many benefits of following the diet. However, it needs to mentioned again, this time as one of the signs that your body is in ketosis. The ketones in your brain provide you with plenty of mental clarity and can help your thought processes. Plus, as you burn off (process) your body's fat stores, you'll notice that you have a lot more energy. Again, once you're in ketosis, you'll experience these things.

As you can see, there are several ways to test to see if you're officially in ketosis. You'll notice changes in the smell of your breath and urine. You can test your blood, along with your breath and urine, using special meters. In addition, you can look for physical and mental signs, including the fact that you look and feel thinner, you have a smaller appetite, and you have a lot more energy and mental clarity. When you examine all of these signs at once, then it will become clear that you're in ketosis.

Chapter #7: Conclusion

Now that you know more about the keto diet, the rest is up to you. If you want to lose weight by burning fat, want to have additional energy and a much clearer mind, then this diet is for you.

What do you need to do next? Choose some of the foods listed in this book, find the best way to track your macros and micros, and get started! Before you know it, you'll have lost that stubborn weight and will feel much better about yourself!